MOST WANTED PLANT BASED DIET COOKBOOK

The ultimate cookbook with easy and tasty recipes to lose weight in a few steps on a budget

Ursa Males

TABLE OF CONTENTS

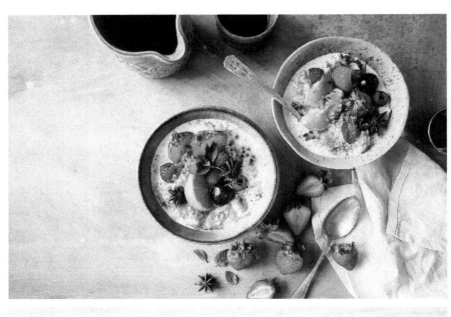

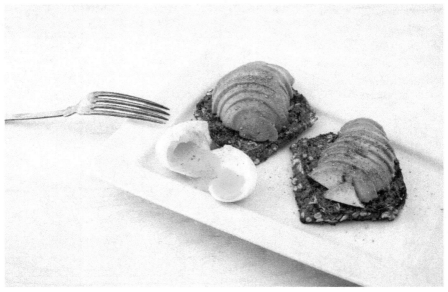

BREAKFAST

1. <u>Almond Hemp Heart Porridge</u>

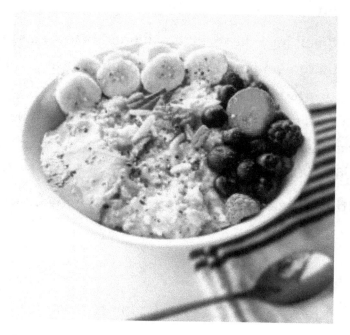

Preparation time: 15 minutes

Cooking time: 5 minutes

Servings: 2

Ingredients:

- ¼ cup almond flour
- ½ tsp cinnamon
- ¾ tsp vanilla extract
- 5 drops stevia

- 1 tbsp chia seeds
- 2 tbsp ground flax seed
- ½ cup hemp hearts
- 1 cup unsweetened coconut milk

Directions:

1. Add all ingredients except almond flour to a saucepan. Stir to combine. Heat over medium heat until it just starts to boil lightly.

2. Once start bubbling, then stir well and cook for 1 minute more. Remove from heat and stir in almond flour. Serve immediately and enjoy.

Nutrition: Calories 329Fat 24.4 g Carbohydrates 9.2 g Protein 16.2 g

2. Cauliflower Zucchini Fritters

Preparation time: 15 minutes

Cooking time: 10 minutes

Servings: 4

Ingredients:

- 3 cups cauliflower florets
- ¼ tsp black pepper
- ¼ cup coconut flour
- 2 medium zucchinis, grated and squeezed
- 1 tbsp coconut oil
- ½ tsp sea salt

Directions:

1. Steam cauliflower florets for 5 minutes. Add cauliflower into the food processor and process until it looks like rice.
2. Add all ingredients except coconut oil to the large bowl and mix until well combined. Make small round patties from the mixture and set them aside.
3. Heat coconut oil in a pan over medium heat. Place patties on pan and cook for 3-4 minutes on each side. Serve and enjoy.

Nutrition: Calories 68 Fat 3.8 g Carbohydrates 7.8 g Protein 2.8 g

3. Chocolate Strawberry Milkshake

Preparation time: 5 minutes

Cooking time: 0 minutes

Servings: 2

Ingredients:

- 1 cup of ice cubes
- ¼ cup unsweetened cocoa powder
- 2 scoops of vegan protein powder
- 1 cup strawberries
- 2 cups unsweetened coconut milk

Directions:

1. Add all fixings into the blender and blend until smooth and creamy. Serve immediately and enjoy.

Nutrition: Calories 221 Fat 5.7g Carbohydrates 15g Protein 27.7 g

4. <u>Ginger Chocolate Oats</u>

Preparation Time: 3 minutes

Cooking time: 0 minutes

Servings: 1

Ingredients:

- 2 tablespoon chocolate chips
- 1 ¾ oz rolled oats
- 1 cup almond milk
- 1 tablespoon cocoa
- 1/2 teaspoon ground ginger
- 1 tablespoon chia seeds
- 1 tablespoon maple syrup

Directions:

1. In a sealable jar or container, place all fixings; put the milk last. Stir the mixture properly and cover. With the jar covered, shake properly to mix the fixings. Keep the jar refrigerated for about 6 hours.

Nutrition: Calories: 347 Carbs: 56g Protein: 17g Fat: 12g

5. Gluten Free Pancakes

Preparation Time: 10 minutes

Cooking time: 5 minutes

Servings: 6

Ingredients:

- 1 cup almond milk, unsweetened
- 1 filled cup cornflour
- 4 teaspoon vanilla extract
- 1 tablespoon baking powder
- 4 teaspoon sugar
- 1/2 teaspoon salt
- Vegan butter

Directions:

1. In a medium bowl, place baking powder, sugar, cornflour, and salt. Using a whisk, mix these Ingredients: properly.
2. Next, add milk and vanilla to the bowl and continue mixing. Place a skillet over medium-low heat—grease pan with vegan butter. Add the contents of your bowl to the skillet, a third of a cup at a time.
3. Cook each side for about 2 minutes. The sides of the pancakes should be set, and bubbles should be noticeable on top.

4. Use a spatula and be gentle when flipping the pancakes. Take them from the pan, and they're ready to serve.

Nutrition: Calories: 95 Carbs: 19g Protein: 1/2g Fat: 1.3

6. <u>Apple Cinnamon Smoothie</u>

Preparation Time: 5 minutes

Cooking time: 0 minutes

Servings: 1

Ingredients:

- 1 tablespoon flaxseed, ground
- 8 oz coconut water
- 1/2 tablespoon protein powder, unsweetened
- 4 raw almonds
- 1 cup apple, diced
- 1 teaspoon vanilla extract
- 1 teaspoon ground cinnamon

Directions:

1. In your blender, add all fixings. Puree for 15 seconds. Pour into a cup and add 3 cubes of ice.

Nutrition: Calories: 238 Carbs: 37.6g Protein: 15.6g Fat: 5g

7. **Pineapple Coconut Mojito Smoothie**

Preparation Time: 5 minutes

Cooking time: 0 minutes

Servings: 1

Ingredients:

- Some ice
- 1 cup coconut milk, unsweetened
- 1 teaspoon chia seeds
- 1/2cup lacinato kale, remove the stems
- 1 tablespoon Sibu Omega-7 Pure
- 1/2 cup spinach leaves, packed
- 1/2-inch piece fresh ginger, peeled
- 1 tablespoon vanilla
- 1/3 cup mint leaves
- 1 cup pineapple chunks, frozen
- 1 lime, peeled, and rind removed

Directions:

1. Put every ingredient except ice in your blender. Puree until a smooth mixture.
2. Add ice cubes and blend once more. Pour into a glass and enjoy.

Nutrition: Calories: 313 Carbs: 30g Protein: 35g Fat: 9g

8. Carrot Cake Quinoa Flake Protein Loaf

Preparation Time: 9 minutes

Cooking time: 6 minutes

Servings: 2

Ingredients:

- 1/2 cup quinoa flakes
- 1/2 cup grated carrots
- 1 1/2 tablespoon protein powder
- 1 teaspoon orange zest
- Pinch salt
- 1/2 cup almond milk, unsweetened
- 4 packets natural sweetener of choice
- 1/3 cup applesauce, unsweetened
- 1 teaspoon ground cinnamon

Directions:

1. In a mini loaf pan, coat with cooking spray. In a medium-sized bowl, add the natural sweeteners, carrots, cinnamon, zest, applesauce, salt, and almond milk. Stir the fixings well.

2. Add protein powder and quinoa flakes. Stir well to incorporate them into the other fixings before putting the entire batter into the loaf pan. Pat the top to make it even.

3. Cook in the microwave within 6 minutes. Your dessert is ready when the top is firm. Set aside to cool before serving.

Nutrition: Calories: 165 Carbs: 26g Protein: 9.5g Fat: 2.5g

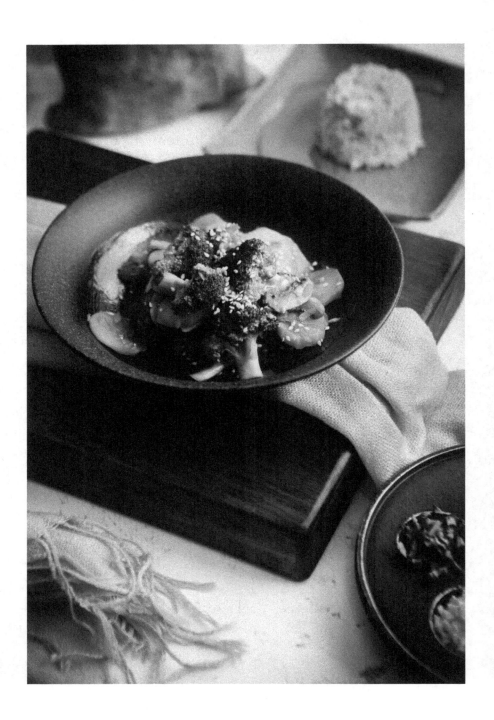

LUNCH

9. Crunchy Rainbow Salad

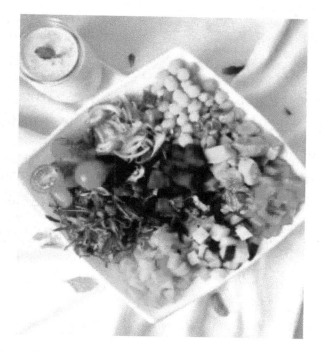

Preparation time: 15 minutes

Cooking time: 0 minutes

Servings: 6

Ingredients:

- 4 cups shredded cabbage, red or green, or bagged slaw mix
- 2 cups cooked edamame

- 1 cup grated or shredded carrots
- ½ bunch cilantro, coarsely chopped
- 2 scallions, thinly sliced
- ½ cup dry roasted peanuts, chopped
- ¾ cup Sweet Peanut Dressing
- Salt

Directions:

1. Combine the cabbage, edamame, carrots, cilantro, scallions, and dry roasted peanuts in a medium bowl and mix well.
2. Add the peanut dressing and mix again, ensuring the dressing is evenly distributed—season with salt to taste.

Nutrition: Calories: 276Fat: 16gCarbohydrate: 21gProtein: 20g

10. **Three-Bean Salad**

Preparation time: 15 minutes

Cooking time: 0 minutes

Servings: 6

Ingredients:

- 1 (14-ounce) can kidney beans, drained & rinsed
- 1 (14-ounce) can chickpeas, drained and rinsed
- 1 (14-ounce) can white navy or cannellini beans, drained and rinsed
- ½ bunch parsley, coarsely chopped
- 2 celery stalks, finely chopped
- 1 red bell pepper, finely chopped
- 1 jalapeño pepper, minced (optional)
- 1 garlic clove, diced (optional)
- ¼ cup apple cider vinegar
- ¼ cup extra-virgin olive oil
- 1 tablespoon Dijon mustard
- 1 tablespoon maple syrup
- ½ teaspoon salt
- Freshly ground black pepper

Directions:

1. Combine the kidney beans, chickpeas, navy beans, parsley, celery, bell pepper, jalapeño pepper, and garlic (if used) in a medium bowl. Mix until evenly combined.

2. Put the apple cider vinegar, olive oil, mustard, maple syrup, and salt into the mixture and add as much black pepper as you'd like. Mix everything thoroughly, taste it, and adjust the seasoning with extra salt, if needed.

Nutrition: Calories: 284Fat: 10gCarbohydrate: 40gProtein: 11g

11. **Greek Salad with Tofu Feta**

Preparation time: 15 minutes

Cooking time: 0 minutes

Servings: 6

Ingredients:

- 1 green bell pepper, coarsely chopped
- 1-pint cherry or grape tomatoes halved
- 1 small red onion, chopped
- 1 cucumber, chopped
- 1 (14-ounce) can butter beans, drained and rinsed
- ½ bunch parsley, coarsely chopped
- ½ cup pitted kalamata olives
- 1 garlic clove, minced
- Juice of 1 lemon
- 3 tablespoons red wine vinegar
- 3 tablespoons olive oil
- Tofu Feta
- 1 teaspoon salt
- Freshly ground black pepper

Directions:

1. In a medium bowl, combine the bell pepper, tomatoes, onion, cucumber, beans, parsley, olives, and garlic. Next, add the lemon juice, vinegar, and oil. Mix well.

2. Add the tofu feta (and any of the tofu marinade) to the salad. Season with salt and as much pepper as you would like, and then mix again.

Nutrition: Calories: 142Fat: 8gCarbohydrate: 14gProtein: 4g

12. Mushroom Lentil Soup

Preparation time: 15 minutes

Cooking time: 40 minutes

Servings: 6

Ingredients:

- 1 tablespoon olive oil
- 1 yellow onion, chopped
- 2 celery stalks, chopped
- 2 carrots, cut into thin rounds
- Pinch + ½ teaspoon salt, divided
- 3 garlic cloves, minced
- 2 cups cremini mushrooms, chopped
- 1 tablespoon dried rosemary
- 6 cups vegetable broth
- 1 cup brown lentils
- 4 cups chopped kale
- 3 tablespoons apple cider vinegar
- Freshly ground black pepper

Directions:

1. In a large stockpot, warm the oil over medium heat. Add the onion, celery, carrots, and a pinch of salt. Cook until the onions are slightly translucent, within 5 minutes.

2. Add the garlic and cook within 1 minute more; then add the mushrooms and rosemary. Stir everything together and cook for 5 minutes more or until the mushrooms have started to release liquid.

3. Add the vegetable broth and lentils. Boil; then reduce the heat to simmer. Cook within 30 minutes or until the lentils have softened. Stir in the kale and allow it to wilt for 1 or 2 minutes more.

4. Add the vinegar, remaining salt, and as much pepper as you'd like. Taste and adjust with additional salt or pepper, if desired.

Nutrition: Calories: 205Fat: 4gCarbohydrate: 27gProtein: 14g

13. **Spicy Peanut Bowl**

Preparation time: 25 minutes

Cooking time: 0 minutes

Servings: 4

Ingredients:

- 1 (8-ounce) package black bean noodles, cooked
- 2 cups cooked edamame beans
- 1 cup red cabbage, thinly sliced
- 1 cup carrots, grated or shredded
- 1 cup red peppers, finely chopped
- 1 cup mung bean or soybean sprouts
- ¼ cup dry roasted peanuts, coarsely chopped
- ¼ cup cilantro, coarsely chopped
- 4 scallions, coarsely chopped
- Sweet Peanut Dressing
- Hot sauce or red chili flakes (optional)

Directions:

1. Divide the noodles evenly among 4 food storage containers. Top each container of noodles with ½ cup of edamame, ¼ cup of cabbage, ¼ cup of carrots, ¼ cup of peppers, ¼ cup of sprouts, and 1 tablespoon of peanuts.

2. Garnish each container with cilantro and scallions. Top it with 3 tablespoons of peanut dressing and hot sauce or chili flakes (if using). Cover the remaining containers with airtight lids and store them in the refrigerator.

Nutrition: Calories: 417Fat: 11gCarbohydrate: 69gProtein: 14g

14. Plant-Strong Power Bowl

Preparation time: 25 minutes

Cooking time: 0 minutes

Servings: 4

Ingredients:

- 2 cups white or brown rice, cooked
- 1 (14-ounce) can of black beans, drained and rinsed
- 1 (14-ounce) can chickpeas, drained and rinsed
- 4 cups spinach, chopped
- 1 cucumber, chopped
- Microgreens, for garnish
- Lemon Parsley Dressing

Directions:

1. Divide the rice evenly among 4 food storage containers, and then add to each container ¼ cup of black beans, ¼ cup of chickpeas, 1 cup of spinach, and ¼ of the chopped cucumber.
2. Garnish each container with a small handful of microgreens. Serve.

Nutrition: Calories: 514Fat: 22gCarbohydrate: 70gProtein: 14g

15. __Burrito Bowl__

Preparation time: 15 minutes

Cooking time: 20 minutes

Servings: 4

Ingredients:

- 1 tablespoon olive oil
- 1 red onion, thinly sliced
- 1 bell pepper, thinly sliced
- Pinch salt
- 1 garlic clove, minced
- ½ teaspoon cumin
- 2 cups white or brown rice, cooked
- 1 (14-ounce) can pinto beans, drained & rinsed
- 4 cups spinach or arugula, chopped
- 1 avocado, chopped
- 4 scallions, coarsely chopped
- Hot sauce or salsa
- Cilantro Lime Dressing

Directions:

1. In a small skillet, warm the oil over medium-high heat. Add the onion, bell pepper, and a big pinch of salt. Sauté for 15 minutes or until the onions begin to

caramelize slightly. Add the garlic and cumin and cook for 3 more minutes. Set aside.

2. Set out 4 food storage containers. To each container, add ½ cup of rice, ¼ of the bell pepper mixture, ¼ cup of beans, 1 cup of greens, and ¼ of the avocado.

3. Garnish each container with scallions and a hot sauce or salsa of your choice.

Nutrition: Calories: 483Fat: 31gCarbohydrate: 50gProtein: 10g

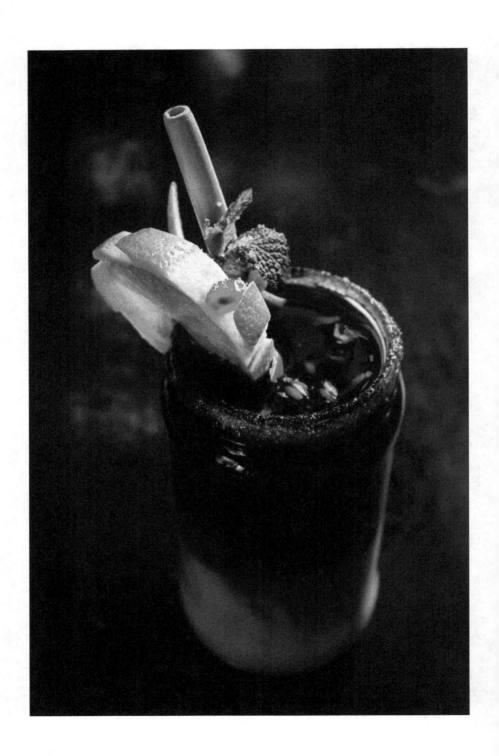

DINNER

16. Cheesy Brussel Sprout Bake

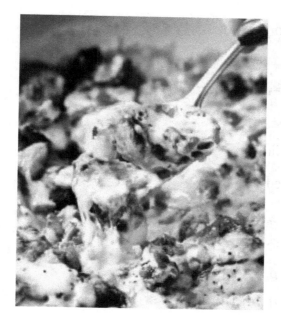

Preparation time: 15 minutes

Cooking time: 46 minutes

Servings: 8

Ingredients:

- ½ onion sliced

2 tbsp. of each:

- garlic, chopped
- avocado oil

- 1 ½ lb. Brussel sprouts

Cheese:

- Dash cayenne

1 tsp of the following:

- onion powder
- salt

¼ tsp of the following:

- pepper
- paprika

½ tsp of the following:

- garlic, powder
- thyme
- 1 tbsp. tapioca starch
- ¼ cup nutritional yeast
- ½ cup vegetable broth
- 1 can coconut cream

Crumble Topping:

- ¼ tsp pepper
- ½ tsp garlic, powder
- 1 tsp salt
- ½ cup panko crumbs

Directions:

1. Bring the oven to 425 heat setting. Prepare Brussel sprouts by washing and trimming then steaming for 10 minutes.

2. Oiled an oven-safe baking dish with nonstick spray. Add the Brussel sprouts to a baking dish and set to the side.

3. Bring a skillet to medium temperature and mix in the garlic, avocado oil, and onion, sautéing approximately 6 minutes. Add the onion mixture to the top of the Brussel sprouts.

4. Put vegetable broth, nutritional yeast, onion powder, pepper, salt, garlic, paprika, thyme, and coconut cream in the same skillet on low heat, whisking together to combine.

5. Carefully add in the tapioca starch and whisk constantly; the mixture will thicken in about 5 minutes. Once it turns into a cheese sauce mixture, pour over the Brussel sprouts and onions.

6. In a mixing container, combine panko, salt, garlic, and pepper, creating the crumble. Sprinkle the crumble across the top of the cheese.

7. Cook in the oven within 25 minutes or until browned and golden. Serve warm and enjoy.

Nutrition: Calories: 116 Carbohydrates: 16 g Proteins: 4 g Fats: 4 g

17. <u>**Caesar Vegan Salad**</u>

Preparation time: 15 minutes

Cooking time: 60 minutes

Servings: 6

Ingredients:

- 5 cups kale, chopped
- 10 cups romaine lettuce

Cheese:

- ½ tsp garlic

1 tbsp. of the following:

- extra virgin olive oil
- nutritional yeast
- 1 garlic clove
- 2 tbsp. hemp seeds, hulled
- 1/3 cup cashews, raw

Caesar Dressing:

½ tsp of the following:

- sea salt
- garlic powder
- Dijon mustard
- 2 tsp capers
- ½ tbsp. vegan Worcestershire sauce

- 2 tbsp. olive oil (best if extra virgin)
- ½ cup raw cashews, soaked overnight
- ¼ cup water
- 1 clove garlic, crushed
- 1 tbsp. lemon juice

Croutons:

- 1/8 tsp cayenne pepper
- ½ tsp of the following:
- garlic powder
- sea salt
- 1 tsp olive oil, (best if extra virgin)
- 14 oz. can chickpeas

Directions:

1. On the day before you plan to make this salad, in a little bowl, soak ½ c. of the raw cashews overnight then drain and rinse.

2. For the croutons, bring the oven to 400 heat setting. Drain the chickpeas and rinse thoroughly. Using a tea towel or cheesecloth, rub the chickpeas so that the skins fall off.

3. Place those in a dish for baking. Spritz the chickpeas with oil and roll them around to coat. Season with cayenne, salt, and garlic powder.

4. Roast the chickpeas for approximately a quarter of an hour or until you are satisfied with the color. Remove from the oven, allowing to cool and become firm.

5. For the dressing, combine everything but not the salt, either in a processor or blender. Blend until smooth liquid consistency.

6. If needed, add ½ tablespoon of water at a time until you have a dressing-like consistency. Season with salt to taste. Set to the side.

7. For the cheese, add garlic and cashews in a food processor, and process them until they reach a finely chopped consistency.

8. Add hemp seeds, nutritional yeast, olive oil, and garlic powder and blend until combined. Season with salt to taste.

9. For the lettuce, after washing the kale, finely chop and set to the side. Chop the lettuce roughly into 2-inch pieces and toss with the kale in a bowl.

10. Pour some dressing and toss again to coat the greens fully. Sprinkle the cheese and croutons over the top. Serve cool and enjoy.

Nutrition: Calories: 284 Carbohydrates: 25.5 g Proteins: 8.7 g Fats: 18.4 g

18. **Mushroom Lettuce Wraps**

Preparation time: 15 minutes

Cooking time: 10 minutes

Servings: 4

Ingredients:

- 8 big leaf romaine lettuce
- 4 green onions, sliced
- ¼ tsp red pepper flakes
- 2 tsp of the following:
- ginger, grated
- canola oil
- 2 cloves garlic
- 12 oz. extra firm tofu
- 1 tsp sesame oil
- 2 tbsp. rice vinegar
- 8 oz. mushrooms, diced
- 1 can water chestnuts
- 3 tbsp. of the following:
- soy sauce, reduced-sodium
- hoisin Sauce

Directions:

1. Whisk together in a little bowl the sesame oil, rice vinegar, soy sauce, and hoisin. Then set to the side.

Open the tofu, and using a paper towel or cheesecloth, remove as much liquid as you can.

2. In a big skillet over medium-high heat, warm the 2 teaspoons of canola oil. Crumble the tofu, making it into little pieces and cook for approximately 5 minutes.

3. Put in the diced mushrooms then cook until almost all the liquid evaporates. Add in the green onions, red pepper, ginger, garlic, and chestnuts and cook for about 30 seconds.

4. Pour the sauce from the little bowl into the skillet and cook until sauce is thoroughly warmed. Plate the individual lettuce leaves and spoon the tofu mixture into each lettuce wrap. Serve and enjoy warm.

Nutrition: Calories: 265 Carbohydrates: 37.6 g Proteins: 13.6 g Fats: 7.9 g

19. <u>**Beefless Stew**</u>

Preparation time: 15 minutes

Cooking time: 50 minutes

Servings: 4

Ingredients:

- 1 tsp dried oregano
- 2 stalks diced celery
- 1 large potato, cubed
- 3 cups sliced carrot
- 2 cups water
- 3 cups vegetable broth
- 1 tsp pepper
- 1 tsp seawater salt
- 2 bulbs mashed garlic
- 1 cup diced onion
- 1 tbsp avocado oil
- bay leaf

Directions:

1. Heat up the avocado oil in an exceeding pot. Put in pepper, salt, garlic cloves, then onion bulbs. Cook everything for 2 to 3 minutes, or until the onion becomes soft.

2. Mix in the bay leaf, oregano, celery, potato, carrot, water, and broth. Allow this to come up to a simmer so that lower the heat down then prepare for 30-45 minutes, or until the carrots and potatoes become soft.

3. Taste and adjust the seasonings that you need to. If it is too thick, you can add some more water or broth. Divide into four bowls and enjoy.

Nutrition: Calories: 238 Carbs: 39g Fat: 4g Protein: 15g

20. **Emmenthal Soup**

Preparation time: 15 minutes

Cooking time: 0 minutes

Servings: 2

Ingredients:

- cayenne
- nutmeg
- 1 tbsp pumpkin seeds
- 2 tbsp chopped chives
- 3 tbsp cubed emmenthal cheese
- 2 cups vegetable broth
- 1 cubed potato
- 2 cups cauliflower pieces

Directions:

1. Place the potato and cauliflower into a saucepan with the vegetable broth just until tender. Place into a blender and puree.
2. Add in spices and adjust to taste. Ladle into bowls, add in chives and cheese and stir well. Garnish with pumpkin seeds. Enjoy.

Nutrition: Calories: 380 Carbs: 0g Fat: 28g Protein: 27g

21. Broccoli "Spaghetti"

Preparation time: 15 minutes

Cooking time: 12 minutes

Servings: 2

Ingredients:

- pepper
- salt
- 1 tsp vegetable broth
- 1 tsp oregano plant
- 1 tbsp juice - lemon
- 3 sliced carrots
- 3 diced tomatoes
- 1 head broccoli cut into floret
- 1 red bell pepper, sliced
- 1 onion bulb, sliced
- 2 diced garlic bulbs, cloves
- 4 tbsp EVOO
- 1 lb. buckwheat pasta

Directions:

1. Place a pot of water on medium and add salt. Allow to boil and add in pasta. Prepare per box instructions. Empty out.

2. Place the broccoli into a different bowl and canopy with water. Prepare for 5 minutes.

3. Put a pan on normal heat and put in two tablespoons of olive oil into the skillet and warm. Put the bulbs, garlic, and onion then prepare till soft and scented. Remove from skillet then set to the side.

4. Add two more tablespoons of olive oil to the skillet and add carrots. Cook for 5 minutes, next put sweet pepper then prepare for another 5 minutes, now put in tomatoes then prepare for 2 minutes.

5. Completely drain the broccoli and add into the skillet with the rest of the vegetables. Put the onions plus garlic back into the skillet.

6. Add vegetable broth, oregano, and lemon juice. Add some pepper and salt, taste and adjust seasonings if needed. Stir well to combine.

7. Place the cooked pasta onto a serving platter. Pour over vegetable mixture and toss to combine.

Nutrition: Calories: 402 Carbs: 60g Fat: 12g Protein: 19g

22. Indian Lentil Curry

Preparation time: 15 minutes

Cooking time: 15 minutes

Servings: 4-6

Ingredients:

- Lime juice
- Chopped cilantro
- Salt
- 1 tbsp EVOO
- 2 Diced tomatoes
- 1 Sliced onion
- 1 clove Minced garlic
- 1-inch Grated ginger
- ½ tsp Turmeric
- ½ tsp Cumin seeds
- 2 Chopped green chilies
- 1 cup Fine red lentils

Directions:

1. Put the lentils into a bowl, fill with water then let sit for 6 hours. After 6 hours, drain the lentils completely.
2. Place a basin on normal warmth. Put in the lentils then cover with fresh water. Allow to boil. Add in turmeric. Lower heat and simmer until lentils are cooked to your

doneness. Pull out from the pot then to a basin. Put these to side.

3. In another pan on medium, warm up olive oil. Add turmeric, cumin, ginger, and onions. Cook until onions are soft and ginger and fragrant. Add chilies and tomatoes, and cook. Add salt and cook for 5 minutes.

4. Pour lentil into this mixture and bring back to a simmer. As shortly it begins to cook, remove it from the hot temperature. Squeeze in some lemon Sprinkle with cilantro and serve with rice.

Nutrition: Calories: 200 Carbs: 24gFat: 1g Protein: 9g

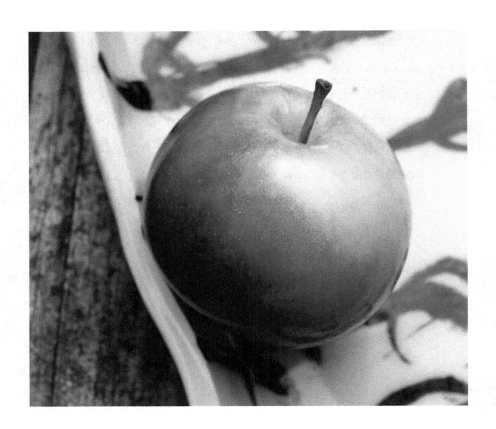

SNACKS

23. Zucchini Muffins

Preparation time: 10 minutes

Cooking time: 30 minutes

Servings: 12

Ingredients:

- 2 cups almond flour
- 2 teaspoons baking powder
- 2 tablespoons coconut sugar
- A pinch of black pepper
- 2 tbsp flaxseed meal + 3 tbsp water, mixed
- ¾ cup almond milk
- 1 cup zucchinis, grated
- ½ cup tofu, shredded

Directions:

1. In a bowl, combine the flour with baking powder, flaxseed and the other ingredients, stir well, divide into a lined muffin tray, introduce in the oven and bake at 400 degrees F for 30 minutes. Serve as a snack.

Nutrition: Calories 149Fat 4gCarbs 14gProtein 5g

24. Nuts and Seeds Squares

Preparation Time: 20 Minutes

Cooking Time: 5 Minutes

Servings: 8

Ingredients:

- ½ cup hazelnuts, toasted
- ½ cup walnuts, toasted
- ½ cup almonds, toasted
- ½ cup white sesame seeds
- ½ cup pumpkin seeds, shelled
- 1 cup unsweetened dried cherries
- 2 cups unsweetened dried coconut flakes
- ¼ cup coconut oil
- 1/3 cup maple syrup
- ½ teaspoon ground cinnamon
- ½ teaspoon salt

Directions:

1. Prepare a 13x9-inch baking dish lined using parchment paper. Set aside. In a large bowl, add the hazelnuts, walnuts, and almonds and mix well.

2. Transfer 1 cup of the nut mixture into another large bowl and chop them roughly. In the food processor,

add the remaining nut mixture and pulse until finely ground.

3. Now, transfer the ground nut mixture into the bowl of the chopped nuts. Add the seeds and coconut flakes and mix well.

4. In a small pan, add the oil, maple syrup, and cinnamon over medium-low heat and cook for about 3–5 minutes or until it starts to boil, stirring continuously.

5. Remove from the heat and immediately pour over the nut mixture, stirring continuously until well combined. Set aside to cool slightly.

6. Now, place the mixture into the prepared baking dish evenly and with the back of a spoon, smooth the top surface by pressing slightly.

7. Refrigerate for about 1 hour or until set completely. Remove from refrigerator and cut into equal sized squares and serve.

Nutrition: Calories: 496Protein: 10gCarbohydrates: 24g

Fat: 42g

25. <u>Seed Bars</u>

Preparation Time: 15 Minutes

Cooking Time: 15 Minutes

Servings: 10

Ingredients:

- 1¼ cups creamy salted peanut butter
- 5 Medjool dates, pitted
- ½ cup unsweetened vegan protein powder
- 2/3 cup hemp seeds
- 1/3 cup chia seeds

Directions:

1. Line a loaf pan with parchment paper. Set aside. In a food processor, add the peanut butter and dates and pulse until well combined.
2. Add the protein powder, hemp seeds, and chia seeds and pulse until well combined. Now, place the mixture into the prepared loaf pan and with the back of a spoon, smooth the top surface.
3. Freeze for at least 10–15 minutes, or until set. Cut into 10 equal sized bars and serve.

Nutrition: Calories: 308Fat: 21gCarbohydrates: 17g

Protein: 16g

26. **Chocolate Protein Bites**

Preparation Time: 10 Minutes

Cooking Time: 20 Minutes

Servings: 12

Ingredients:

- ½ cup Chocolate Protein Powder
- 1 Avocado, medium
- 1 tbsp. Chocolate Chips
- 1 tbsp. Almond Butter
- 1 tbsp. Cocoa Powder
- 1 tsp. Vanilla Extract
- Dash of Salt

Directions:

1. Begin by blending avocado, almond butter, vanilla extract, and salt in a high-speed blender until you get a smooth mixture.
2. Next, spoon in the protein powder, cocoa powder, and chocolate chips to the blender. Blend again until you get a smooth dough-like consistency mixture.
3. Now, check for seasoning and add more sweetness if needed. Finally, with the help of a scooper, scoop out dough to make small balls.

Nutrition: Calories: 46Fat: 2gCarbohydrates: 2gProtein: 2g

27. __Spicy Nuts and Seeds Snack Mix__

Preparation Time: 5 Minutes

Cooking Time: 10 Minutes

Servings: 4

Ingredients:

- ¼ tsp garlic powder
- ¼ tsp nutritional yeast
- ½ tsp smoked paprika
- ¼ tsp sea salt
- ¼ tsp dried parsley
- ½ cup slivered almonds
- ½ cup cashew pieces
- ½ cup sunflower seeds
- ½ cup pepitas

Directions:

1. Mix the garlic powder, nutritional yeast, paprika, salt, and parsley in a small bowl. Set aside. In a large skillet, add the almonds, cashews, sunflower seeds, pepitas and heat over low heat until warm and glistening, 3 minutes.

2. Turn the heat off and stir in the parsley mixture. Allow complete cooling and enjoy!

Nutrition: Calories: 385Fat: 33gProtein: 12g Carbohydrates: 16g

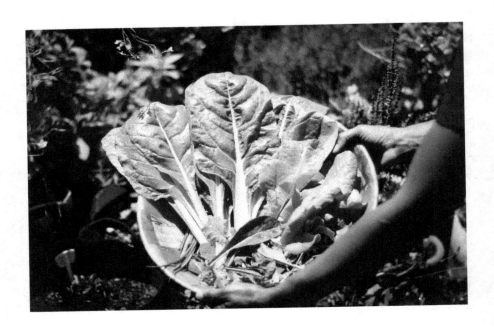

VEGETABLES

28. Potato Latke

Preparation Time: 15 minutes

Cooking Time: 10 minutes

Servings: 6

Ingredients:

- 3 eggs, beaten
- 1 onion, grated
- 1 ½ teaspoons baking powder
- Salt and pepper to taste
- 2 lb. potatoes, peeled and grated
- ¼ cup all-purpose flour
- 4 tablespoons vegetable oil
- Chopped onion chives

Direction

1. Prep your oven to 400 degrees F.
2. Scourge eggs, onion, baking powder, salt and pepper.
3. Squeeze moisture from the shredded potatoes using paper towel.
4. Add potatoes to the egg mixture.
5. Stir in the flour.

6. Fill oil into a pan over medium heat.
7. Cook a small amount of the batter for 3 to 4 minutes per side.
8. Repeat. Garnish with the chives.

Nutrition: 266 Calories 34.6g Carbohydrates 7.6g Protein

29. **Broccoli Rabe**

Preparation Time: 15 minutes

Cooking Time: 15 minutes

Servings: 8

Ingredients:

- 2 oranges, sliced in half
- 1 lb. broccoli rabe
- 2 tablespoons sesame oil, toasted
- Salt and pepper to taste
- 1 tablespoon sesame seeds, toasted

Direction

1. Fill oil into a pan over medium heat.
2. Add the oranges and cook until caramelized.
3. Transfer to a plate.
4. Put the broccoli in the pan and cook for 8 minutes.
5. Squeeze the oranges to release juice in a bowl.
6. Stir in the oil, salt and pepper.
7. Coat the broccoli rabe with the mixture.
8. Sprinkle seeds on top.

Nutrition: 59 Calories 4.1g Carbohydrates 2.2g Protein

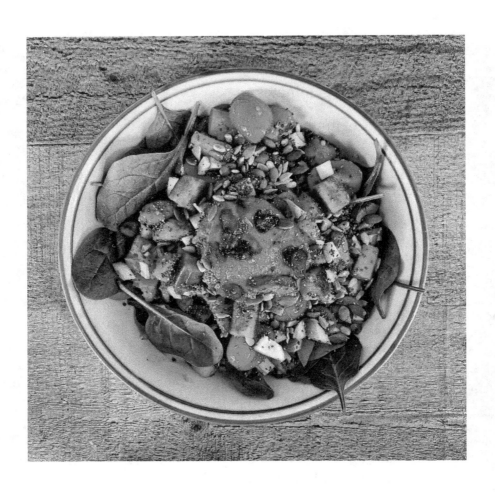

SALAD

30. Potato Tuna Salad

Preparation Time: 4 hours and 20 minutes

Cooking Time: 10 minutes

Servings: 6

Ingredients:

- Water
- 3 potatoes, peeled and sliced into cubes
- ½ cup plain yogurt
- ½ cup mayonnaise
- 1 clove garlic, crushed and minced
- 1 tablespoon almond milk
- 1 tablespoon fresh dill, chopped
- ½ teaspoon lemon zest
- Salt to taste
- 1 cup cucumber, chopped
- ¼ cup scallions, chopped
- ¼ cup radishes, chopped
- 9 oz. canned tuna flakes
- 2 hard-boiled eggs, chopped
- 6 cups lettuce, chopped

Instructions:

1. Fill your pot with water.
2. Add the potatoes and boil.
3. Cook for 10 minutes or until slightly tender.
4. Drain and let cool.
5. In a bowl, mix the yogurt, mayo, garlic, almond milk, fresh dill, lemon zest and salt.
6. Stir in the potatoes, tuna flakes and eggs.
7. Mix well.
8. Chill in the refrigerator for 4 hours.
9. Stir in the shredded lettuce before serving.

Nutrition: Calories 243 Fat 9.9 g Saturated fat 2 g

Carbohydrates 22.2 g Fiber 4.6 g Protein 17.5 g

31.   **Shrimp Veggie Pasta Salad**

Preparation Time: 50 minutes

Cooking Time: 10 minutes

Servings: 6

Ingredients:

- 1 lb. shrimp, peeled and deveined
- 8 oz. asparagus, sliced
- Salt and pepper to taste
- 12 oz. farfalle, penne or macaroni pasta, cooked
- 2 tablespoons parsley, chopped
- ½ cup shallots, sliced thinly
- ¼ cup Parmesan cheese, grated
- 2 tablespoons freshly squeezed lemon juice
- ½ cup mayonnaise
- 2 teaspoons garlic, minced
- 1 teaspoon Worcestershire sauce
- 1 teaspoon Dijon mustard
- 1 lemon, sliced into wedges

Instructions:

1. Preheat your oven to 400 degrees F.
2. Arrange the shrimp and asparagus in a baking pan.
3. Season with the salt and pepper.
4. Roast in the oven for 10 minutes.

5. Let cool. Transfer to a bowl.

6. Stir in the cooked pasta, parsley and shallots.

7. Sprinkle the Parmesan cheese on top.

8. In another bowl, combine the lemon juice, mayonnaise, garlic, Worcestershire sauce and Dijon mustard.

9. Add this mixture to the pasta salad.

1. Toss to coat evenly.

2. Refrigerate for at least 30 minutes before serving.

3. Garnish with the lemon wedges.

Nutrition: Calories 429 Fat 17.1 g Saturated fat 2.8 g

Carbohydrates 45.6 g Fiber 7.2 g Protein 25 g

GRAINS

32. Coconut Chickpea Curry

Preparation Time: 5 minutes

Cooking Time: 15 minutes

Servings: 4

Ingredients:

- 2 tsps. coconut flour
- 16 oz. cooked chickpeas
- 14 oz. tomatoes, diced
- 1 red onion, sliced
- 1 ½ tsps. minced garlic
- ½ tsp. sea salt
- 1 tsp. curry powder
- 1/3 tsp. ground black pepper
- 1 ½ tbsps. garam masala
- ¼ tsp. cumin
- 1 lime, juiced
- 13.5 oz. coconut milk, unsweetened
- 2 tbsps. coconut oil

Directions:

1. Take a large pot, place it over medium-high heat, add oil and when it melts, add onions and tomatoes, season with salt and black pepper and cook for 5 minutes.
2. Switch heat to medium-low level, cook for 10 minutes until tomatoes have released their liquid, then add chickpeas and stir in garlic, curry powder, garam masala, and cumin until combined.
3. Stir in milk and flour, bring the mixture to boil, switch heat to medium heat and simmer the curry for 12 minutes until cooked.
4. Taste to adjust seasoning, drizzle with lime juice, and serve.

Nutrition: Calories: 225, Fat: 9.4 g ,Carbs: 28.5 g, Protein: 7.3 g

33. **Cauliflower Steak with Sweet-pea Puree**

Preparation Time: 5 minutes

Cooking Time: 30 minutes

Servings: 2

Ingredients:

Cauliflower:

- 2 heads cauliflower
- 1 tsp. olive oil
- ¼ tsp. Paprika
- 1 tsp. Coriander
- ¼ tsp. Black pepper

Sweet-pea puree:

- 10 oz. frozen green peas
- 1 onion, chopped
- 2 tbsps. fresh parsley
- ¼ c. unsweetened soy milk

Directions:

1. Preheat oven to 425F.
2. Remove bottom core of cauliflower. Stand it on its base, starting in the middle, slice in half. Then slice steaks about ¾ inches thick.
3. Using a baking pan, set in the steaks.
4. Using olive oil, coat the front and back of the steaks.

5. Sprinkle with coriander, paprika, and pepper.

6. Bake for 30 minutes, flipping once.

7. Meanwhile, steam the chopped onion and peas until soft.

8. Place these vegetables in a blender with milk and parsley and blend until smooth.

Nutrition: Calories 234, Fat 3.8g, Carbs 40.3g, Protein 14.5g

LEGUMES

34. Hot and Spicy Anasazi Bean Soup

Preparation Time: 10 minutes

Cooking Time: 10 minutes

Servings: 4

Ingredients:

- 2 cups Anasazi beans, soaked overnight, drained and rinsed
- 8 cups water
- 2 bay leaves
- 3 tablespoons olive oil
- 2 medium onions, chopped
- 2 bell peppers, chopped
- 1 habanero pepper, chopped
- 3 cloves garlic, pressed or minced
- Sea salt and ground black pepper, to taste

Directions

1. In a soup pot, bring the Anasazi beans and water to a boil. Once boiling, turn the heat to a simmer. Add in the bay leaves and let it cook for about 1 hour or until tender.

2. Meanwhile, in a heavy-bottomed pot, heat the olive oil over medium-high heat. Now, sauté the onion, peppers and garlic for about 4 minutes until tender.

3. Add the sautéed mixture to the cooked beans. Season with salt and black pepper.

4. Continue to simmer, stirring periodically, for 10 minutes more or until everything is cooked through. Bon appétit!

Nutrition: Calories: 352; Fat: 8.5g; Carbs: 50.1g; Protein: 19.7g

BREAD & PIZZA

35. <u>Broccoli Bread</u>

Preparation Time: 10 Minutes

Cooking Time: 30 Minutes

Servings: 5

Ingredients:

- Eggs – 5, lightly beaten
- Broccoli florets – 3/4 cup, chopped
- Cheddar cheese – 1 cup, shredded
- Baking powder – 2 teaspoons.
- Coconut flour – 3 1/1 tablespoons.
- Salt – 1 teaspoon.

Directions:

1. Preheat the oven to 350 F. Grease loaf pan with butter and set aside. Add all Ingredients into the bowl and mix well.
2. Pour egg mixture into the prepared loaf pan and bake for 30 minutes.
3. Slice and serve.

Nutrition: Calories 205,Carbs 8g, Fat 13g, Protein 13g

36. <u>Tasty Tomato Garlic Mozzarella Pizza</u>

Preparation time: 20 minutes

Cooking time: 2 hours 30 minutes

Servings: 6

Ingredients:

- 12 inch of frozen whole-wheat pizza crust, thawed
- 3/4 teaspoon of tapioca flour
- 2 teaspoons of minced garlic
- 2 teaspoons of agar powder
- 1 teaspoon of cornstarch
- 1 teaspoon of salt, divided
- 1/2 teaspoon of red pepper flakes
- 1/2 teaspoon of dried basil
- 1/2 teaspoon of dried parsley
- 2 tablespoons of olive oil
- 1/4 teaspoon of lemon juice
- 3/4 teaspoon of apple cider vinegar
- 8 fluid ounce of coconut milk, unsweetened

Directions:

1. Start by preparing the mozzarella.
2. Place a small saucepan over a medium-low heat, pour in the milk and let it steam until it gets warm thoroughly.

3. With a whisker, pour in the agar powder and stir properly until it dissolves completely.
4. Switch the temperature to a low and pour in the salt, lemon juice, vinegar, and whisk them properly.
5. Mix the tapioca flour and cornstarch with 2 tablespoons of water before adding it to the milk mixture.
6. Whisk properly and transfer this mixture to a greased bowl.
7. Place the bowl in a refrigerator for 1 hour or until it is set.
8. Then grease a- 4 to 6 quarts of the slow cooker with a non-stick cooking spray and insert pizza crust into it.
9. Press the dough into the bottom and brush the top with olive oil.
10. Spread the garlic and then cover it with the tomato slices.
11. Sprinkle it with salt, red pepper flakes, basil, and the oregano.
12. Cut the mozzarella cheese into coins and place them across the top of the pizza.
13. Cover it with the lid, plug in the slow cooker, let it cook for 1 to 1 1/2 hours at the low heat setting or until the crust turns golden brown and the cheese melts completely.

14. When done, transfer the pizza to the cutting board, then let it rest for 5 minutes, and slice to serve.

Nutrition: Calories: 113 Cal, Carbohydrates: 10g, Protein: 7g, Fats: 5g, Fiber: 1g.

SOUP AND STEW

37. **Amazing Chickpea and Noodle Soup**

Preparation Time: 10 minutes

Cooking Time: 20 minutes

Servings: 1 cup

Ingredients:

- 1 freshly diced celery stalk
- ¼ cup of 'chicken' seasoning
- 1 cup of freshly diced onion
- 3 cloves of freshly crushed garlic
- 2 cups of cooked chickpeas
- 4 cups of vegetable broth
- Freshly chopped cilantro
- 2 freshly cubed medium-size potatoes
- Salt
- 2 freshly sliced carrots
- ½ teaspoon of dried thyme
- Pepper
- 2 cups of water
- 6 ounces of gluten-free spaghetti
- 'Chicken' seasoning

- 1 tablespoon of garlic powder
- 2 teaspoons of sea salt
- 1 1/3 cup of nutritional yeast
- 3 tablespoons of onion powder
- 1 teaspoon of oregano
- ½ teaspoon of turmeric
- 1 ½ tablespoons of dried basil

Directions:

1. Put a pot on medium heat and sauté the onion. It will soften within 3 minutes.
2. Add celery, potato, and carrots and sauté for another 3 minutes
3. Add the 'chicken' seasoning to the garlic, thyme, water, and vegetable broth.
4. Simmer the mix on medium-high heat. Cook the veggies for about 20 minutes until they soften.
5. Add the cooked pasta and chickpeas.
6. Add salt and pepper to taste.
7. Put the fresh cilantro on top and enjoy the fresh soup!

Nutrition: kcal: 405 Carbohydrates: 1 g Protein: 19 g Fat: 38 g

38. __Lentil Soup the Vegan Way__

Preparation Time: 5 minutes

Cooking Time: 20 minutes

Servings: 1 cup

Ingredients:

- 2 tablespoons of water
- 4 stalks of thinly sliced celery
- 2 cloves of freshly minced garlic
- 4 thinly sliced large carrots
- Sea salt
- 2 freshly diced small shallots
- Pepper
- 3 cups of red/yellow baby potatoes
- 2 cups of chopped sturdy greens
- 4 cups of vegetable broth
- 1 cup of uncooked brown or green lentils
- Fresh rosemary/thyme

Directions:

1. Put a large pot over medium heat. Once the pot is hot enough, add the shallots, garlic, celery, and carrots in water. Season the veggies with a little bit of pepper and salt.

2. Sauté the veggies for 5 minutes until they are tender. You will know that the veggies are ready when they have turned golden brown. Be careful with the garlic, because it can easily burn.

3. Add the potatoes and some more seasoning. Cook for 2 minutes.

4. Mix the vegetable broth with the rosemary. Now Increase the heat to medium-high. Allow the veggies to be in a rolling simmer. Add the lentils and give everything a thorough stir.

5. Once it starts to simmer again, decrease the heat and simmer for about 20 minutes without a cover. You will know that the veggies are ready when both the lentils and potatoes are soft

6. Add the greens. Cook for 4 minutes until they wilt. You can adjust the flavor with seasonings.

7. Enjoy this with rice or flatbread. The leftovers are equally tasty, so store them well to enjoy on a day when you are not in the mood to cook.

Nutrition: kcal: 284 Carbohydrates: 21 g Protein: 11 g Fat: 19 g

SAUCES, DRESSINGS & DIP

39. Tasty Ranch Dressing/Dip

Preparation time: 45 minutes

Cooking time: 45 minutes

Servings: 16

Ingredients:

- 1/2 c. soy milk, unsweetened
- 1 tablespoon dill, chopped
- 2 t. parsley, chopped
- 1/4 t. black pepper
- 1/2 t. of the following:
- Onion powder
- Garlic powder
- 1 c. vegan mayonnaise

Directions:

1. In a medium bowl, whisk all the **Ingredients:** together until smooth. If dressing is too thick, add 1/4 tablespoon of soy milk at a time until the desired consistency.

2. Transfer to an airtight container or jar and refrigerate for 1 hour.

3. Serve over leafy greens or as a dip.

Nutrition: Calories: 93 Carbohydrates: 0 g Proteins: 0 g Fats: 9 g

40. <u>Creamy Avocado Cilantro Lime Dressing</u>

Preparation Time: 5 minutes

Cooking Time: 0 minutes

Servings: 2

Ingredients:

- 1 avocado, diced
- ½ cup water
- ¼ cup cilantro leaves
- ¼ cup fresh lime or lemon juice (about 2 limes or lemons)
- ½ teaspoon ground cumin
- ¼ teaspoon salt (optional)

Directions:

1. Put all the ingredients in a blender (high-speed blenders work best for this), and pulse until well combined. Taste and adjust the seasoning as needed. It is best served within 1 day.

Nutrition: calories: 94fat: 7.4g carbs: 5.7gprotein: 1.1g fiber: 3.5g

APPETIZER

41. <u>Marinated Mushroom Wraps</u>

Preparation time: 15 minutes

Cooking time: 0 minutes

Servings: 2

Ingredients:

- 3 tablespoons soy sauce
- 3 tablespoons fresh lemon juice
- 1½ tablespoons toasted sesame oil
- 2 portobello mushroom caps, cut into 1/4-inch strips
- 1 ripe Hass avocado, pitted and peeled
- 2 (10-inch) whole-grain flour tortillas
- 2 cups fresh baby spinach leaves
- 1 medium red bell pepper, cut into ¼ inch strips
- 1 ripe tomato, chopped
- Salt and freshly ground black pepper

Directions:

1. In a medium bowl, combine the soy sauce, 2 tablespoons of the lemon juice, and the oil. Add the portobello strips, toss to combine, and marinate for 1 hour or overnight.

2. Drain the mushrooms and set aside. Mash your avocado with the remaining 1 tablespoon of lemon juice.

3. To assemble wraps, place 1 tortilla on a work surface and spread with some of the mashed avocado. Top with a layer of baby spinach leaves.

4. In the lower third of each tortilla, arrange strips of the soaked mushrooms and some of the bell pepper strips.

5. Sprinkle with the tomato and salt and black pepper to taste. Roll up tightly and cut in half diagonally. Repeat with the remaining Ingredients and serve.

Nutrition: Calories: 112 Carbs: 5g Fat: 7g Protein: 1g

42. Tamari Toasted Almonds

Preparation time: 2 minutes

Cooking time: 8 minutes

Servings: ½ cup

Ingredients:

- ½ cup raw almonds, or sunflower seeds
- 2 tablespoons tamari, or soy sauce
- 1 teaspoon toasted sesame oil

Directions:

1. Heat a dry skillet to medium-high heat, then add the almonds, stirring frequently to keep them from burning.
2. Once the almonds are toasted—7-8 minutes for almonds, or 34 minutes for sunflower seeds—pour the tamari and sesame oil into the hot skillet and stir to coat.
3. You can turn off the heat, and as the almonds cool the tamari mixture will stick and dry on to the nuts.

Nutrition: Calories: 89Fat: 8gCarbs: 3gProtein: 4g

43. Avocado and Tempeh Bacon Wraps

Preparation time: 10 minutes

Cooking time: 8 minutes

Servings: 4

Ingredients:

- 2 tablespoons extra-virgin olive oil
- 8 ounces tempeh bacon, homemade or store-bought
- 4 (10-inch) soft flour tortillas or lavash flat bread
- ¼ cup vegan mayonnaise, homemade or store-bought
- 4 large lettuce leaves
- 2 ripe Hass avocados, pitted, peeled, and cut into ¼-inch slices
- 1 large ripe tomato, cut into ¼-inch slices

Directions:

1. Heat-up the oil in a large skillet over medium heat. Add the tempeh bacon and cook until browned on both sides, about 8 minutes. Remove from the heat and set aside.

2. Place 1 tortilla on a work surface. Spread with some of the mayonnaise and one-fourth of the lettuce and tomatoes.

3. Thinly slice the avocado and place the slices on top of the tomato. Add the reserved tempeh bacon and roll up tightly. Repeat with remaining Ingredients and serve.

Nutrition: Calories: 315 Carbs: 22g Fat: 20g Protein: 14g

SMOOTHIES AND JUICES

44. Banana Milk

Preparation time: 5 minutes

Cooking time: 0 minute

Servings: 2

Ingredients:

- 2 dates
- 2 medium bananas, peeled
- 1 teaspoon vanilla extract, unsweetened
- 1/2 cup ice
- 2 cups of water

Directions:

1. Place all the ingredients in the order in a food processor or blender and then pulse for 2 to 3 minutes at high speed until smooth.
2. Pour the smoothie into two glasses and then serve.

Nutrition: Calories: 79 Cal Fat: 0 g Carbs: 19.8 g Protein: 0.8 g Fiber: 6 g

45.   Apple, Carrot, Celery and Kale Juice

Preparation time: 5 minutes

Cooking time: 0 minute

Servings: 2

Ingredients:

- 5 curly kale
- 2 green apples, cored, peeled, chopped
- 2 large stalks celery
- 4 large carrots, cored, peeled, chopped

Directions:

1. Process all the ingredients in the order in a juicer or blender and then strain it into two glasses.
2. Serve straight away.

Nutrition: Calories: 183 Cal Fat: 2.5 g Carbs: 46 g Protein: 13 g Fiber: 3 g

DESSERTS

46. <u>Apple Crisp</u>

Preparation time: 15 minutes

Cooking time: 40 minutes

Servings: 6

Ingredients:

- ½ cup vegan butter
- 6 large apples, diced large
- 1 cup dried cranberries
- 2 tablespoons granulated sugar
- 2 teaspoons ground cinnamon, divided
- ¼ teaspoon ground nutmeg
- ¼ teaspoon ground ginger
- 2 teaspoons lemon juice
- 1 cup all-purpose flour
- 1 cup rolled oats
- 1 cup brown sugar
- ¼ teaspoon salt

Directions:

1. Preheat the oven to 350°F. Oiled an 8-inch square baking dish with butter or cooking spray.

2. Make the filling. In a large bowl, combine the apples, cranberries, granulated sugar, 1 teaspoon of cinnamon, the nutmeg, ginger, and lemon juice. Toss to coat. Transfer the apple mixture to the prepared baking dish.

3. Make the topping. In the same large bowl, now empty, combine the all-purpose flour, oats, brown sugar, and salt. Stir to combine.

4. Add the butter and, using a pastry cutter (or two knives moving in a crisscross pattern), cut the butter into the flour and oat mixture until the butter is the size of small peas.

5. Spread the topping over the apples evenly, patting down slightly. Bake for 40 minutes or until golden and bubbly.

Nutrition: Calories: 488Fat: 9 g Carbs: 101 g Protein: 5 g

47. **Secret Ingredient Chocolate Brownies**

Preparation time: 15 minutes

Cooking time: 35 minutes

Servings: 6-8

Ingredients:

- ¾ cup flour
- ¼ teaspoon baking soda
- ¼ teaspoon salt
- 1/3 cup vegan butter
- ¾ cup sugar
- 2 tablespoon water
- 1¼ cups semi-sweet or dark dairy-free chocolate chips
- 6 tablespoons aquafaba, divided
- 1 teaspoon vanilla extract

Directions:

1. Preheat the oven to 325°F. Line a 9-inch square baking pan with parchment or grease well. In a large bowl, combine the flour, baking soda, and salt. Set aside.

2. In a medium saucepan over medium-high heat, combine the butter, sugar, and water. Bring to a boil, stirring occasionally. Remove then stir in the chocolate chips.

3. Whisk in 3 tablespoons of aquafaba until thoroughly combined. Add the vanilla extract and the remaining 3 tablespoons of aquafaba, and whisk until mixed.

4. Add the chocolate mixture into the flour mixture and stir until combined. Pour in an even layer into the prepared pan.

5. Bake for 35 minutes, until the top is set but the brownie jiggles slightly when shaken. Allow to cool completely, 45 minutes to 1 hour, before removing and serving.

Nutrition: Calories: 369Fat: 19 g Carbs: 48 g Protein: 4 g

48. Chocolate Chip Pecan Cookies

Preparation time: 15 minutes

Cooking time: 16 minutes

Servings: 30 cookies

Ingredients:

- ¾ cup pecan halves, toasted
- 1 cup vegan butter
- ½ teaspoon salt
- ½ cup powdered sugar
- 2 teaspoons vanilla extract
- 2 cups all-purpose flour
- 1 cup mini dairy-free chocolate chips, such as Enjoy Life brand

Directions:

1. Preheat the oven to 350°F. Prepare a large rimmed baking sheet lined using parchment paper.
2. In a small skillet over medium heat, toast the pecans until warm and fragrant, about 2 minutes. Remove from the pan. Once these are cool, chop them into small pieces.
3. Combine the butter, salt, and powdered sugar, and cream using an electric hand mixer or a stand mixer fitted with a paddle attachment on high speed for 3 to 4

minutes, until light and fluffy. Add the vanilla extract and beat for 1 minute.

4. Turn the mixer on low and slowly add the flour, ½ cup at a time, until a dough form. Put the chocolate chips plus pecans, and mix until just incorporated.

5. Using your hands, a large spoon, or a 1-inch ice cream scoop, drop 1-inch balls of dough on the baking sheet, spaced 1 inch apart. Gently press down on the cookies to flatten them slightly.

6. Bake for 12 to 14 minutes until just golden around the edges. Cool on the baking sheet within 5 minutes before transferring them to a wire rack to cool. Serve or store in an airtight container.

Nutrition: Calories: 152Fat: 11 g Carbs: 13 g Protein: 2 g

49. Peanut Butter Chip Cookies

Preparation time: 15 minutes

Cooking time: 15 minutes

Servings: 12-15

Ingredients:

- 1 tablespoon ground flaxseed
- 3 tablespoons hot water
- 1 cup rolled oats
- 1 teaspoon baking soda
- 1 teaspoon ground cinnamon
- ¼ teaspoon salt
- 1 ripe banana, mashed
- ¼ cup maple syrup
- ½ cup all-natural smooth peanut butter
- 1 tablespoon vanilla extract
- ½ cup dairy-free chocolate chips

Directions:

1. Preheat the oven to 350°F. Prepare a large rimmed baking sheet lined using parchment paper.
2. Make a flaxseed egg by combining the ground flaxseed and hot water in a small bowl. Stir and let it sit for 5 minutes until thickened.

3. In a medium bowl, combine the oats, baking soda, cinnamon, and salt. Set aside.

4. Mash the banana then put the maple syrup, peanut butter, flaxseed egg, and vanilla extract in a large bowl. Stir to combine.

5. Add the dry batter into the wet batter and stir until just incorporated (do not overmix). Gently fold in the chocolate chips.

6. Using a large spoon or 2-inch ice cream scoop, drop the cookie dough balls onto the baking sheet. Flatten them slightly.

7. Bake within 12 to 15 minutes or until the bottoms and edges are slightly browned. Serve or store in an airtight container.

Nutrition: Calories: 192Fat: 12 g Carbs: 17 g Protein: 6 g

50. <u>No-Bake Chocolate Coconut Energy Balls</u>

Preparation time: 15 minutes

Cooking time: 0 minutes

Servings: 9

Ingredients:

- ¼ cup dry roasted or raw pumpkin seeds
- ¼ cup dry roasted or raw sunflower seeds
- ½ cup unsweetened shredded coconut
- 2 tablespoons chia seeds
- ¼ teaspoon salt
- 1½ tablespoons Dutch process cocoa powder
- ¼ cup rolled oats
- 2 tablespoons coconut oil, melted
- 6 pitted dates
- 2 tablespoons all-natural almond butter

Directions:

1. Combine the pumpkin seeds, sunflower seeds, coconut, chia seeds, salt, cocoa powder, and oats in a food processor or blender. Pulse until the mix is coarsely crumbled.

2. Add the coconut oil, dates, and almond butter. Pulse until the batter is combined and sticks when squeezed between your fingers.

3. Scoop out 2 tablespoons of mix at a time and roll them into 1½-inch balls with your hands. Place them spaced apart on a freezer-safe plate and freeze for 15 minutes.

4. Remove from the freezer and keep refrigerated in an airtight container for up to 4 days.

Nutrition: Calories: 230Fat: 12 g Carbs: 27 g Protein: 5 g